The Thinki Surviva to Managing a Menopausal PARTNER

CW01019979

TIGGY BAILEY

Published by Clink Street Publishing 2022

Copyright © 2022

First edition.

ISBNs:
978-1-915229-57-1 Paperback
978-1-915229-58-8 Ebook

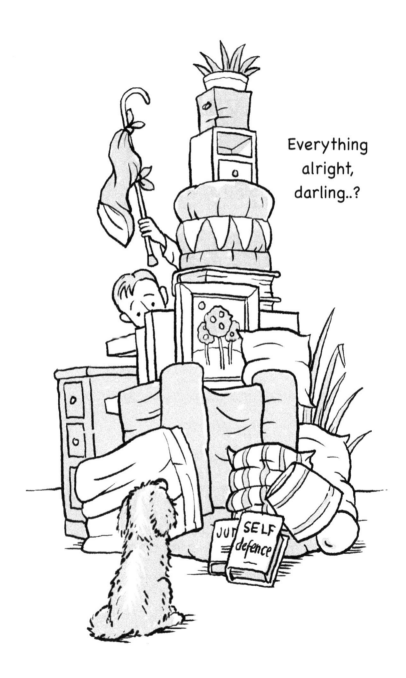

First and most important principle:

At all times deny categorically that you have even noticed any suggestion whatsoever that your significant other may be experiencing menopausal symptoms.

This will carry you a long way, and even, some of the time, with a following wind, render some of the principles detailed here unnecessary.

It is a brave man, however, who will take this on trust.

Believe you me, there is a very large gap between men and women, and, dare I say it, even more between men and menopausal women.

Men are from Mars and women are from Venus, or so it's been said.

Well of course, for menopausal women are hot and nearer the sun!

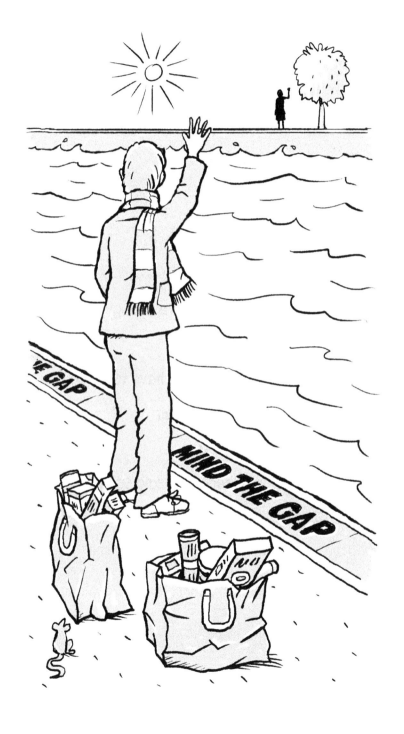

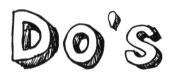 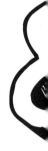

Do

Always think you're wrong

✓

Obey orders even when to have to do so is

grossly unfair

✓

Understand "because I said so" is a

valid reason

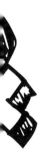

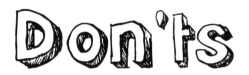 Don'ts

Don't

Ever think you're right – even when you are

✗

Refuse to obey orders, even when to obey

would be akin to suicide

✗

Offer to shut that window

✗

Expect pleases and thank yous

✗

Comment on the bed linen being changed

again, even midweek

Mood Management for the Gentleman

Maintain a placid and acquiescent air at all times.

Beware however that occasionally this will be perceived to be sycophantic and patronising.

You will not be able to predict when this will occur.

There will be times to be masterful and commanding, but it will be impossible to know when these are.

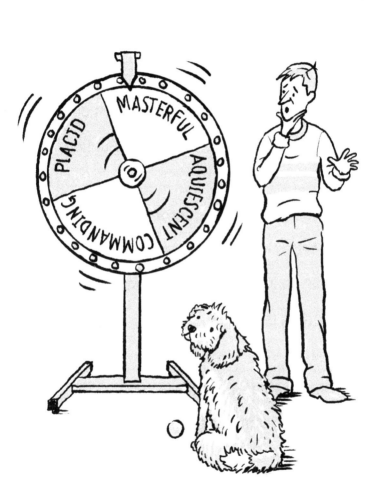

Mood swings in the lady

Beware sudden outbursts of emotion out of all proportion to the instigating situation.

Just go with it if she cries when Liv in *Made in Chelsea* has had a row with her boyfriend, or the neighbours hang their washing in an upsetting manner.

If she's furious with you, just accept you will have done something suitably bad to justify this rage.

Like wear the wrong colour T-shirt or stack the dishwasher in the wrong order.

Don't ever enrage her further by apologising, or worse still, ask what you've done wrong.

Whatever you do, don't do that. It should be obvious.

If she's furious with someone else, agree wholeheartedly that they are a terrible person and deserve to be hated and to be treated like a pariah.

Be careful however as when they abruptly cease to be persona non grata for no obvious discernible reason and becomes her best friend again, you will be in trouble for so outrageously and unfairly slagging them off.

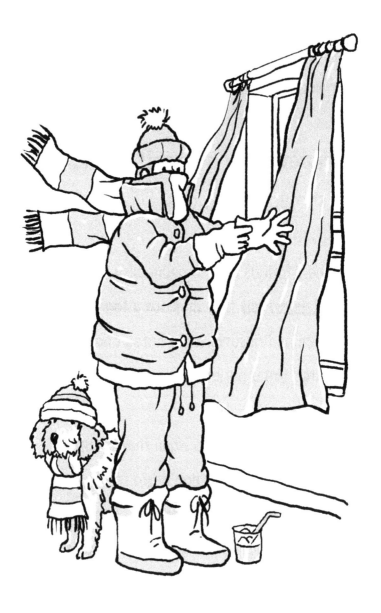

Temperature management

Never presume to say, "It's a bit chilly in here isn't it?" even if it would freeze the nipples off a brass monkey.

Just quietly add another layer, or put on a winter coat, gloves and scarf, and man up.

<u>Never mention:</u>

HRT

•

The oestrogenic principles of soya

•

"Perhaps an appointment with the GP might
be helpful"

•

Weight gain

•

Fluid retention, cellulite, puffy ankles, cankles,
saddle bags, or bingo wings, even on other
women. Except Gwyneth Paltrow. Slag her off
at every available opportunity

•

Vagisil (other brands are available)

<u>Gifts to avoid:</u>

Cosmetic surgery

•

Elastic waisted garments, however practical

•

Wrinkle cream

•

Any TENA Lady products

(other brands are available)

•

Vagisil

Day to day management

Silence is not the way to respond to rants or even seemingly placidly uttered statements, however oft heard.

This will only enrage and lead to even more repetition.

Instead, greet these statements or rants with careful acknowledgement.

Blanket agreement, which makes it obvious that you weren't actually listening, not only won't help but will just enrage, or enrage further.

Pick carefully from the points she is making and use one of these in your response.

This will stand you in great stead as a good listening ear, and on-side, achieving Brownie Points that may well be very useful, nay necessary, on other occasions when you have unwittingly transgressed.

Beware:

Brownie Points cannot be stored and redeemed at a later date.

Yes, we are aware of the contradiction here.

Get over it.

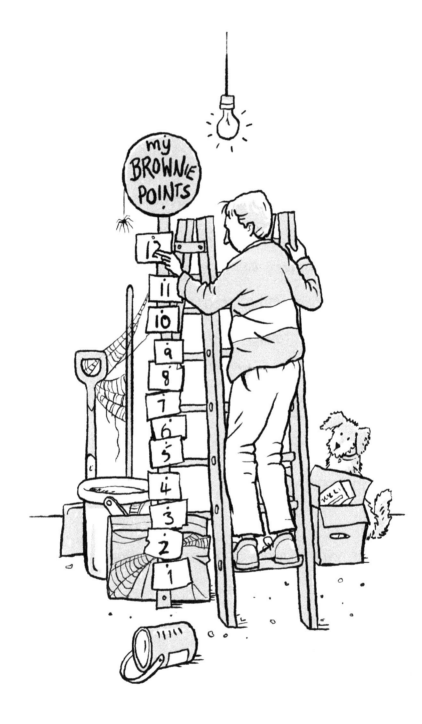

Saying **"Whaaaaat?"**

in what you believe to be an amusing yet
gently questioning tone, will not ingratiate
you in any way.

Nor will it get you out of trouble when you
have failed to respond in a way that is
deemed adequate.

You may think zoning out a good coping
strategy.

It is not.

Arguments

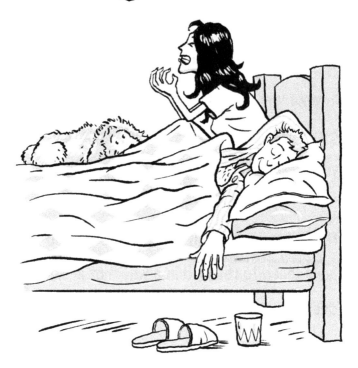

More likely to happen than
pre-menopausally.

Don't ask if that is indeed a word.

Just accept that it is.

"Never go to bed on an argument," is the truest of expressions, you just can't imagine how true.

The problem is knowing when that argument has satisfactorily been dealt with.

You may think your point has been well made, accepted, and the argument is over.

You will then fall asleep and sleep the sleep of the righteous.

You boys are good at that.
Your lady is not.

See comments about insomnia in two chapters' time.

You may well wake up in a lovely sunny mood, last night having been completely forgotten.

My goodness how you will suffer.

Your sunny mood will vanish like a puff of smoke when her grumpiness and her banging on about the awful night's sleep she had, which was all your fault, lead to a day of total misery for you.

The argument will be dragged back up in spades, embellished and expanded upon in ways you never imagined.

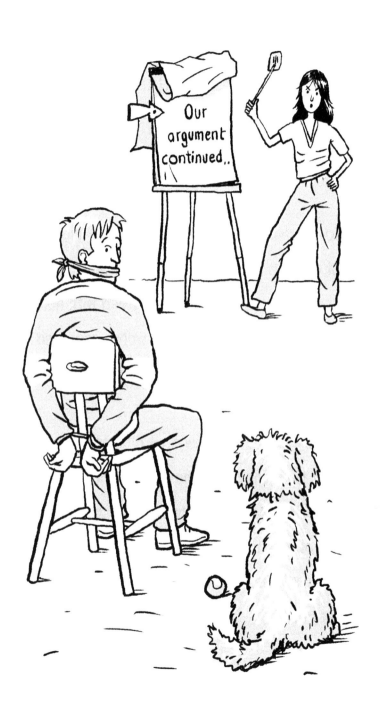

If I were you, I'd find an excuse to go out somewhere, in fact anywhere.

To prevent this, accept that the lady's idea of an argument being resolved is when you have absolutely and totally agreed with her point of view, in the correct words, repeated several times, in a very convincing manner.

Otherwise she will stew on it all night, go over what she should have said, what you should have said, totally make mountains out of molehills, plan all sorts of revenge; and you'll just end up having to agree with her anyway.

You might just as well follow the correct route of resolution (whilst quietly knowing that you are right really), and get it over with.

Don't ever voice this inner knowledge out loud or the whole thing will just roll out again.

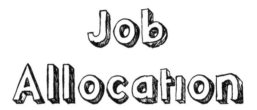

Job Allocation

Beware job requests from your menopausal partner.

There may seem to be a yawning gulf between what the lady actually asks and what the lady actually means.

For example:

"Is the dishwasher full?"

To the gentleman, this may seem to be an innocuous and simple closed question requiring a simple yes / no answer.

So far from the truth!

What it actually means is, "Please can you
see if the dishwasher is full, and if not, fill it
(remembering the point above about how
easily wrath can be incurred by incorrectly
stacked dishwashers), put a tablet in, check
the rinse aid and the salt, turn it on and
be prepared to empty it again when the
programme has finished."

Remember to select the correct
programme.

This will depend on whether your partner is in
"economy" mode or "thorough cleaning of
everything" mode.

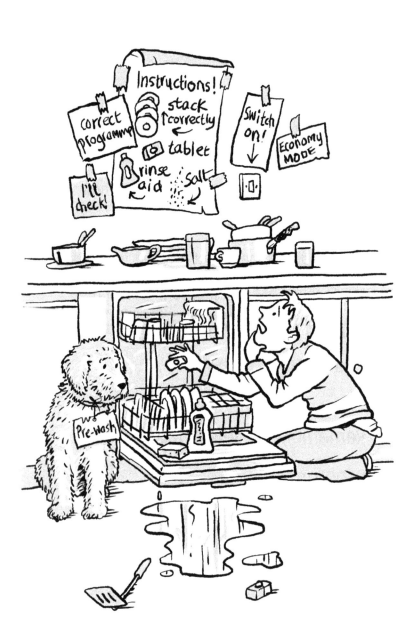

Selecting the wrong programme and failing to match the correct mode will not go down well.

If the dishwasher tablets are anything below half in The Required Supply, add dishwasher tablets to the shopping list.

Likewise rinse aid and dishwasher salt.

A second example:

"Please could you get the ironing board out?"

Woe betide any gentleman who just gets the ironing board out. So very very wrong sir!

What it actually means is, "Please get the ironing board out, and the iron, turn it on to warm up on the approved setting, fetch the ironing from wherever to-be-done ironing is being collected.

Preferably actually do the ironing. That would be much appreciated."

Just getting the ironing board out will go down like a plate of vomit and you will suffer accordingly.

Statements of protestation such as "I thought you wanted it for..." will fall on deaf ears.

Don't waste your breath.

Warning:

lobbing something any-old-how into a cupboard so it is merely out of sight is not putting something away!

Insomnia

A common problem in the menopausal lady. Beware any nocturnal behaviours such as, god forbid, snoring.

A heinous behaviour indeed.

When ladies snore, that is not their fault, they hate the fact that they snore and of course it must not be stated out loud that they do so.

If ever mentioned it should be commented that it is in fact "charming" and "lovely to know you're getting well deserved rest darling."

When the gentleman snores on the other hand, it is a very different matter.

It is done to vex and annoy and the gentleman must desist.

If this means the wearing of cumbersome devices that preclude sleep, well too bad – now you'll appreciate the sufferings of the insomniac too.

Being woken up or pummelled or punched when you're keeping the lady awake with your snoring is perfectly fair.

You must just suck this up.

Reciprocation is not fair however, I refer you back to the comment on the previous page.

Think carefully on the timing of talking, even if whispering sweet nothings, and of cuddles and caresses as these may arouse the lady just as she is drifting off.

And not in a good way.

You will not be thanked.

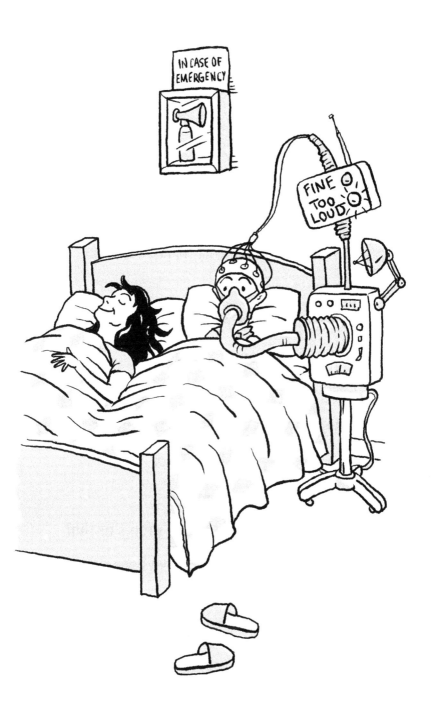

Observations

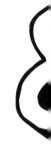

<u>Be warned:</u> the lady, particularly the menopausal lady, will have a phenomenal memory for certain things, such as:-

Anything you've ever said that might be deemed derogatory

•

Anything you've ever said that might be deemed critical

•

Anything you've ever done wrong, or that has been perceived to have been done incorrectly, or insufficiently

You may not have shared that perception.

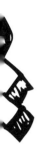

Recollections

Be warned also: the lady, particularly the menopausal lady, will have a phenomenal ability to forget certain things, such as:–

Any compliments you may have paid her

•

Any nice things you have done for her

•

All the many things that you have done correctly, even in the rare event that you've managed to do them correctly in her perception. Likely as rare as hen's teeth, especially if they were done at the right time too.

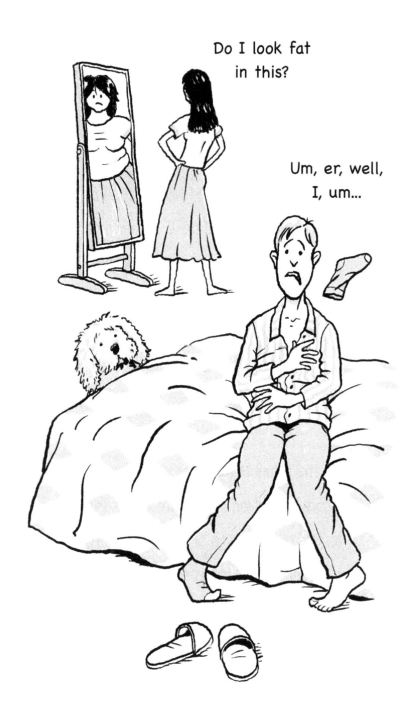

If asked, "Do I look fat in this?" Do not look!

Male logic may suggest you can't give an objective opinion without assessment. An objective opinion is not required and an appraising look will not be welcomed.

It means you are considering that she might indeed look fat in that.

You may think preventing the lady in question going out in an outfit that makes her looks like the stern of the QE2 would be a good thing.

All your tact and diplomacy are required here.

"You look lovely darling" – purely sarcastic.

"You always look lovely darling, whatever you're wearing" – even more sarcastic.

"Perhaps your blue dress will be more suitable today, you don't want to outshine the hostess" might work.

On some occasions.

But you can only use such a thing once, so save it for a very special moment.

There will be times when simply nothing will work and you will cause upset one way or another.

No point wasting your carefully considered most diplomatic lines here.

Best just to accept whatever punishment is meted out to you and live to fight another day.

The age question! Oh be so careful here! It is not quite so dangerous as the "Do I look fat?" question, but not far off.

Embrace the concept of the white lie for self-preservation reasons. If you are asked how old your partner looks, take off ten years from her real age.

Any more, and she won't believe you to be genuine.

Any less and she will be insulted.

If you are asked how old another lady is,
by that other lady herself, take at least ten
years off the age you think she is.

**Hopefully she will trot off,
flattered and happy.**

The next bit is very critical however. You must
avoid being seen to be paying compliments
to another lady, even if she is a very good
friend.

Your significant other will immediately think
she looks much older than the other lady
in your opinion; and worse, also much older
than she actually is.

(All the insomnia and the hormonal issues may mean this is in fact true, but truth hurts, especially the vulnerable menopausal lady).

Pick your moment most carefully.

As soon as you are out of earshot of the third party, whisper lovingly to your partner "I only said that to be polite, 'X' looks much older than you, darling. Much, much older. You don't look a day over_____"
(Insert appropriately flattering age here).

Practise a believable tone in anticipation of such occasions.

OCDs

All ladies are prone to such things, particularly the menopausal one.

You may not share, understand or even wish to tolerate a behaviour that seems ludicrous to you, but it will be well worth your while to do so. Double electric switches having to have both switches pointing the same way is a perfectly normal thing. Using clothes pegs colour coordinated to the clothing pegged with them is not a quirk, it makes for a tidy clothesline. The neighbours might be looking.

It doesn't matter that she disapproves of the way that they hang their washing. That is irrelevant.

The loo seat!

In theory, the rule is that it should be left
as it is found. Rather like countryside gates.
That is what shall be proclaimed if asked.
But please be aware that it should be found
with the seat down, the lid not open, and
absolutely categorically not with the seat up.

The left up loo seat shall incur great
wrath. For there may have been splashes
or sprinkles. Ladies don't like to think of such
things and wish to believe gentlemen sit
down to avoid any such risk.

Your aim may not be as good as
you think.

No wonder the menopausal lady might seem to have a "tweezer fetish". You chaps might not mind hair no longer growing where it should and it sprouting in profusion where it shouldn't, but menopausal ladies do.

Those bristly chin hairs must be attacked within a microsecond of their discovery, or she simply can't concentrate on anything else.

Yes this does explain why there is a pair of tweezers in the car. And in every travel bag. And in fact near every well lit mirror. Best not to draw attention to this fact or the tweezers might be redirected your way, at those inviting protruding nose hairs for example, that are just screaming to be plucked.

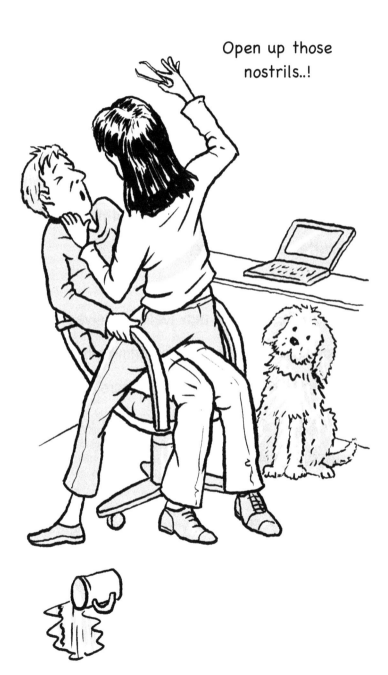

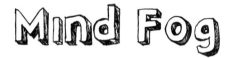

Mind Fog

Yes, chaps, this is indeed a thing!

It is not just an excuse for absentmindedness, inattention or apparent insults.

Menopausal ladies may feel themselves to be operating through an obfuscating mist, even though previously their minds were as sharp as a knife and quick as mercury (or so they liked to think).

Do not be offended if your beloved addresses you with the dog's name, or perhaps that of another human.

This does not mean the dog occupies a more important mind-space than you, nor that your partner is having an affair with the other named person.

It is merely likely that recall is affected by Mind Fog.

I stress, please do not be insulted.

After all the dog, or that other person, might be a being it is a compliment to be mistaken for.

Best to pretend that you haven't even noticed.

Lists

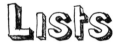

Lists are a necessity of life, especially if the compiler tends in any way towards a blue personality. (That is blue as in DISC Colour Profiling rather than blue in mood, though of course both might apply). Only when there are lists of lists should you be concerned that it is going too far.

Lists allow a sense of achievement which is very important for the menopausal lady, who is likely to have issues with self-worth. Things may even be written on the list even when they've been done already, just so they can be crossed off. A nice long list, all ticked off, is a thing of beauty.

And a thing of beauty is a joy forever.

In Summary

Best advice for the gentleman sharing his world with a menopausal partner is perhaps to accept that you can't do right for doing wrong.

Life's a bitch and all that.

Keep your head down, survive, and pray supplies of HRT from China get back to matching demand.

There will be clear sunlit times ahead.

One day!

Ooh a pig flew past...